Kama S

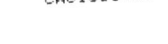

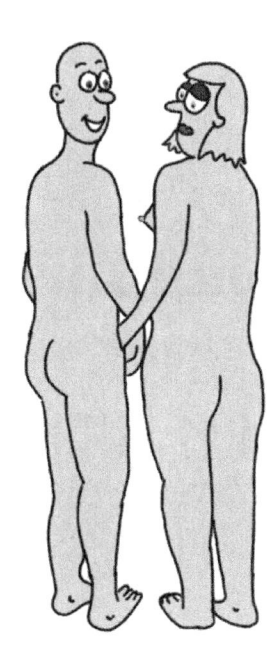

With

Bob and Brenda

CONTAINS ADULT IMAGES

Written and Illustrated
By
Paul Gwilliam

Also available
Bob and Brenda's Joke Book

Disclaimer

Bob and Brenda are not responsible for any injuries you may
sustain while attempting anything shown in this book.
So don't be a knob head. Be careful.

Introduction

Hello and welcome to our Kama Sutra book. We hope you're going to have as much fun reading this book as we have had making it.

We don't want to bore you with the history of Kama Sutra, let's just say it's from India, it's many years old and it's Rude.

Our Kama Sutra book contains illustrations and instructions to different sex positions that you can add to your love making sessions.

It's just a bit of fun and not meant to be taken too seriously.

So, buy a bottle of wine, turn the lights down low, put your Barry White CD on and start your journey into the world of the Kama Sutra.

Bob and Brenda

A Word About Safe Sex

Practise safe sex and you're less likely to pick up a Sexually Transmitted Infection, HIV or get pregnant.
You must use condoms. Sex and condoms go together like Bob and Brenda. You can't have one without the other.

Remember: More partners means bigger risks.
So, have fun but please be careful.
For more information please search the web.

Thank you.

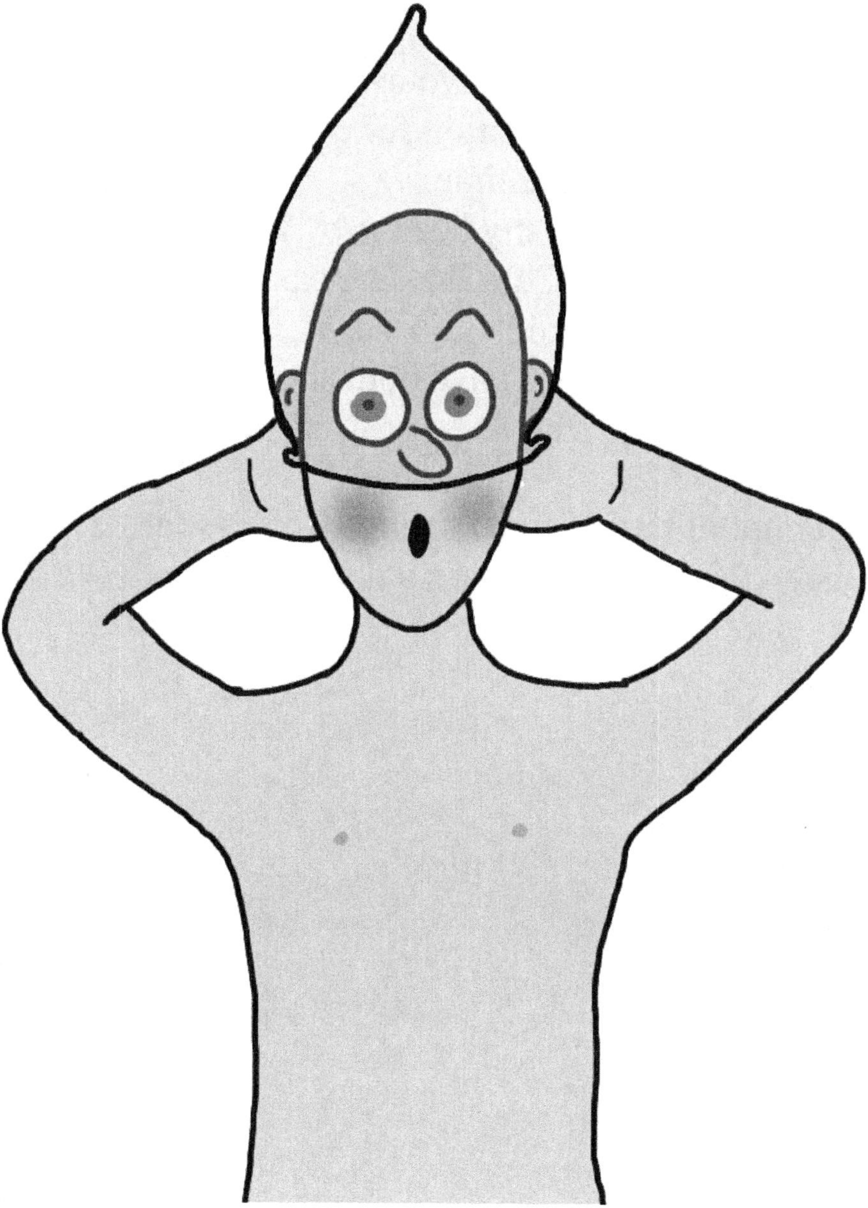

69

Ok, let's start with Bob's favourite.

The 69 is the perfect position for us to satisfy each other orally at the same time.

We lie side by side so my head is by Bob's willy and Bob's head is by my Cha Cha. We can then start oralling (Is that a word?).

We must make sure we have both showered and our bum holes are poo free.

Lost count of the amount of times Bob has farted whilst in this position. That's a definite no-no.

Brenda

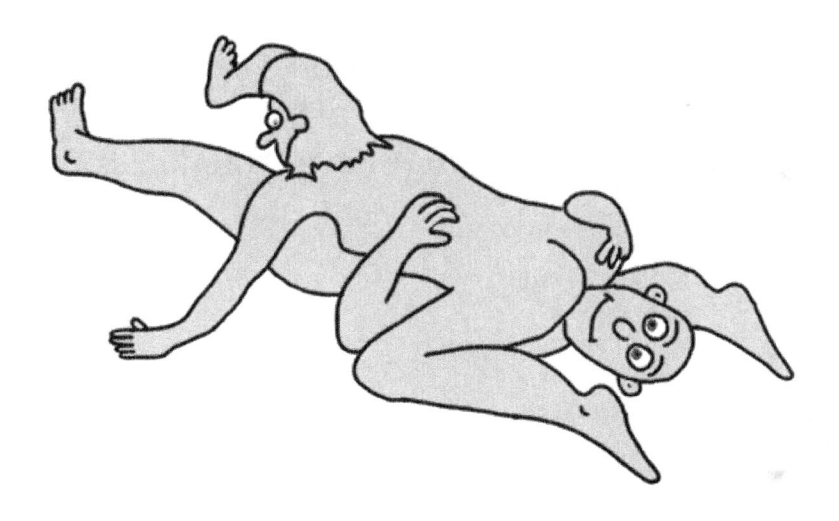

Afternoon Delight

Afternoon, Day or Night Delight. Who cares when? I like this one when done on the stairs before going upstairs to our love nest.

Brenda sits on the stair or end of the bed, I kneel down between her legs and enter her La La with my Dipsy. We have good eye contact with this position and Brenda can snog my face off.
No eating garlic beforehand.
You may need skateboard pads on your knees.... It helps.

Bob

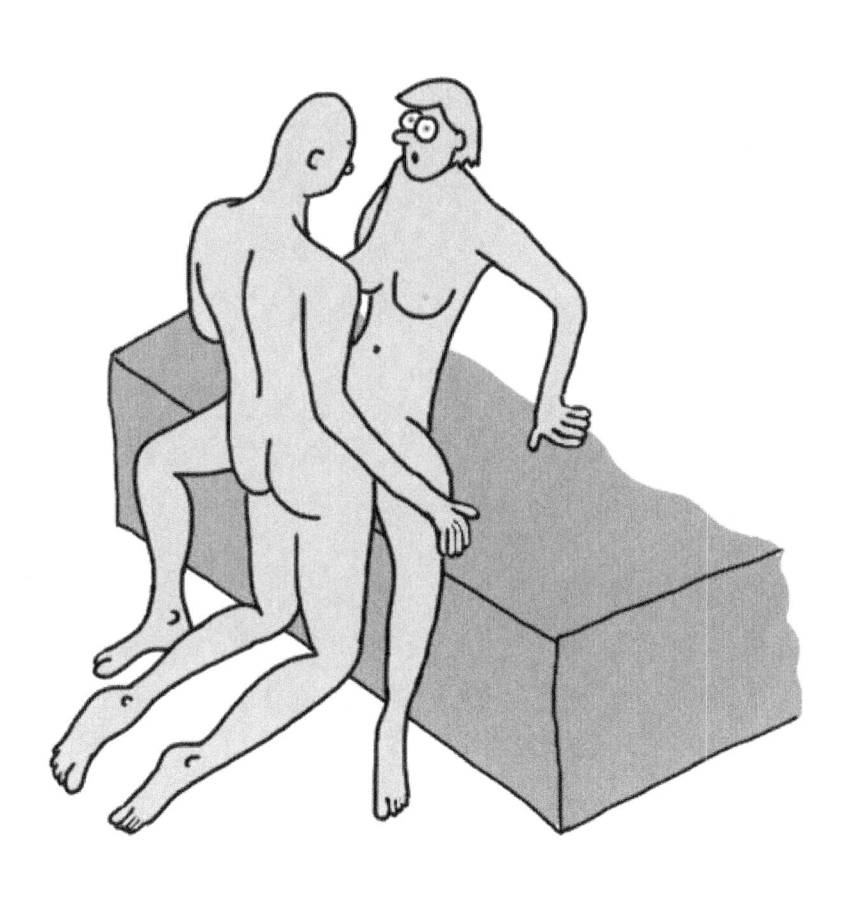

Amazon

I know what you're thinking 'online shopping site' but you would be so wrong.
I like this position because I get to sit down. Lol

Bob lies down and brings his knees up to his chest. His manhood peeks out like a meerkat. I sit on Bob so his meerkat enters my burrow.

Simples....

Brenda

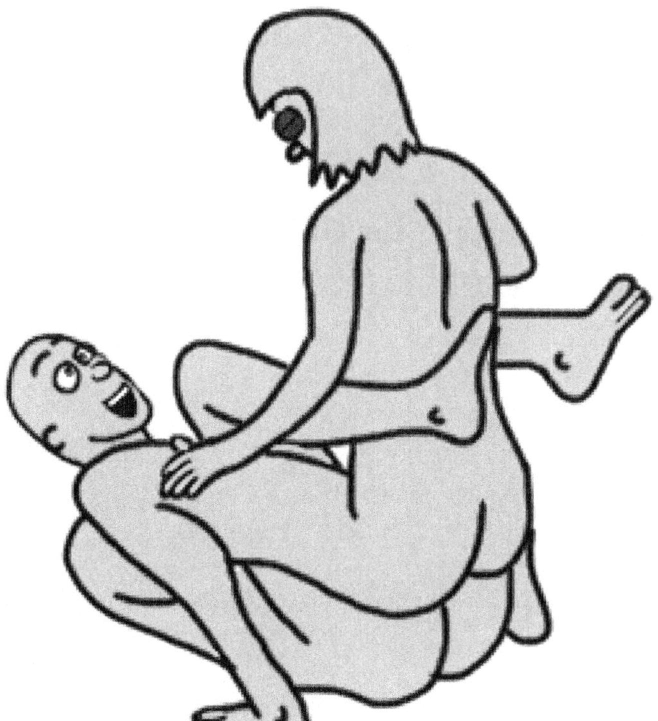

Arch

Feeling fit? No? Maybe this position isn't for you then.

Brenda lies on the floor and lifts her bum and back up using her legs. I kneel between her legs and insert my coin into her slot.

I enjoy this position because I have a good view of Brenda's boobs and I can flick her fanny nose with my thumb. Lol

This is a great exercise for Brenda's belly muscles....and one of the reasons she looks so good.

Bob

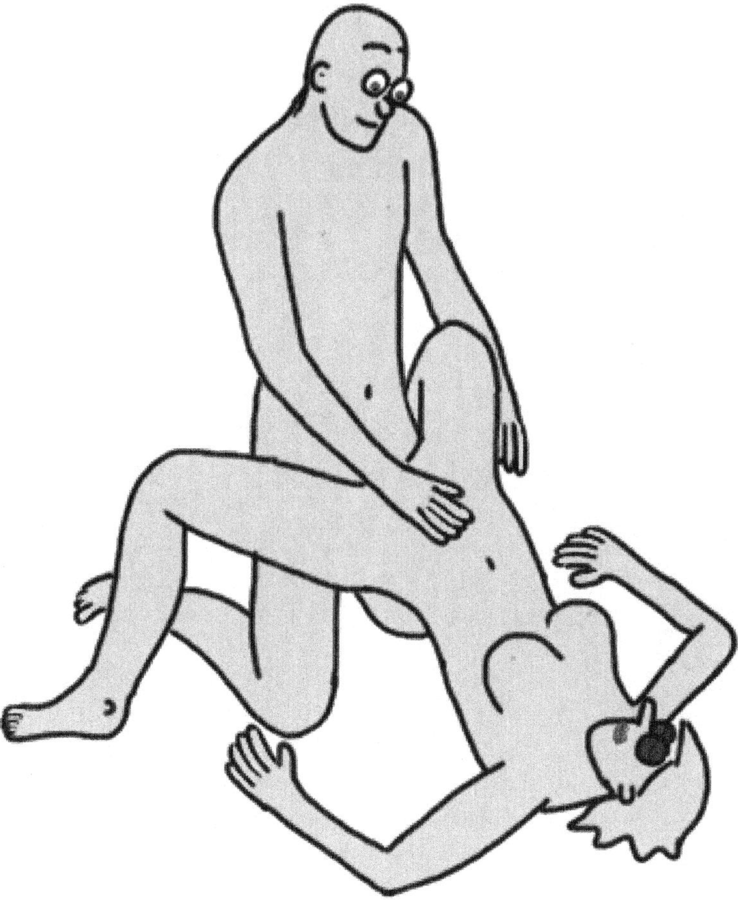

Atten-Hut

Stand to attention and get your wobbler out Bob. Lol This is an easy one. I kneel down in front of Bob and put his wobbler in my mouth.

I give him great oral sex in the hope that his legs will give way and he will fall in a heap on the floor. When we're both feeling a bit more adventurous I reach round with my hand and stick my finger up his bum while I'm giving him head....He likes that.

Brenda

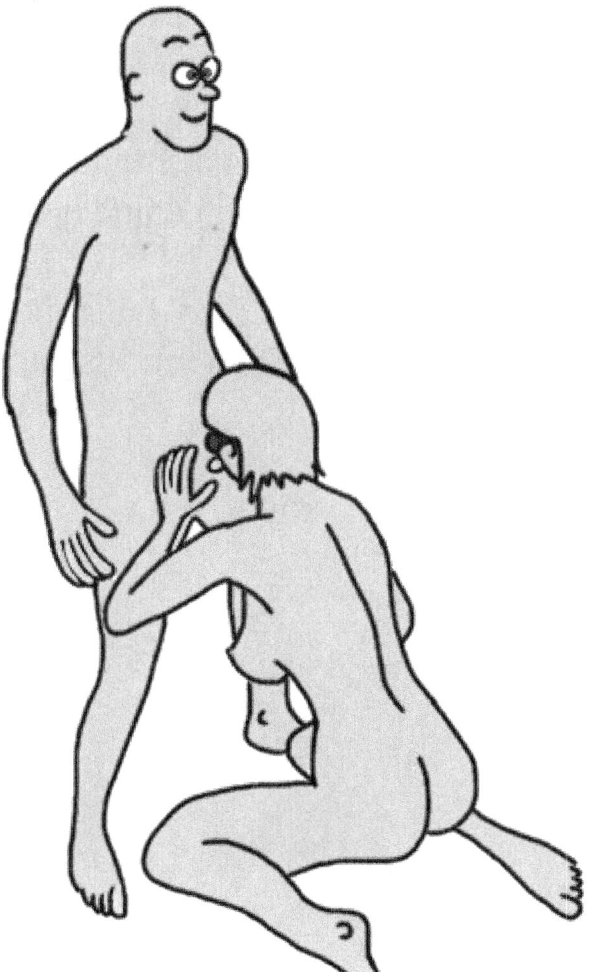

Ben Dover

"Right Brenda, bend over and touch your toes."
"Okay babe...Ooooooooo."

Simple one this. Brenda bends over and touches her toes (No shit Sherlock). I stand behind her and put my Mop in her Bucket.
I also get a good view of her dirty bullet hole and if she agrees I insert my finger into it. Instant poo finger.

Mmmmmm love this position.

Bob

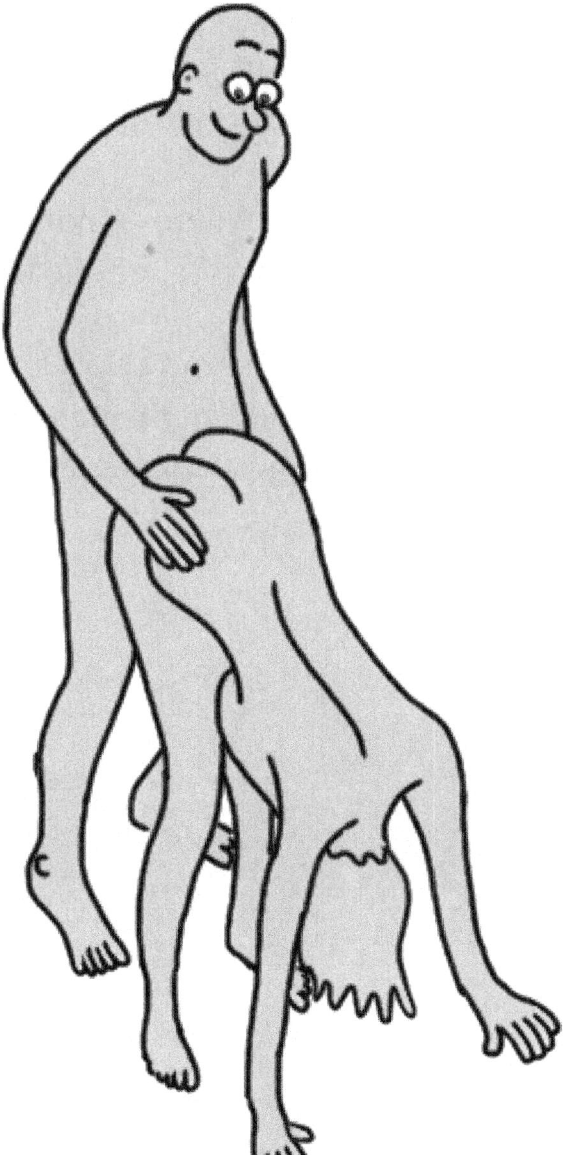

Blow Job

I think everybody's heard of a Blow Job, No! it's not something you do in a Balloon factory. It's simply the act of putting your cheese stick in your girlfriends mouth.
It can be done almost anywhere, driving the car, in the elevator, sitting on the sofa, on the toilet or in the supermarket.

I like to lie flat on my back and watch while Brenda gives me a Blow Job. Makes me feel like a lazy king.

Go Brenda go...

Bob

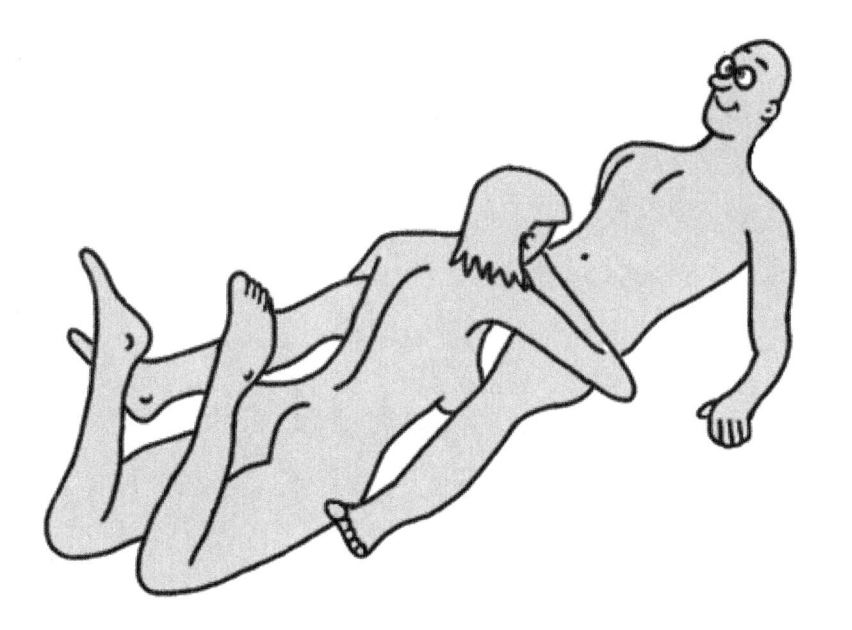

Bodyguard

"And I...I....will always love you...Ooooooooo" Lol

I think this is called the bodyguard because Bob protects my behind with his little soldier.
I like to reach round with both my arms and clench his bum cheeks.

Bob gets a good feel of my Fun bags too.

Brenda

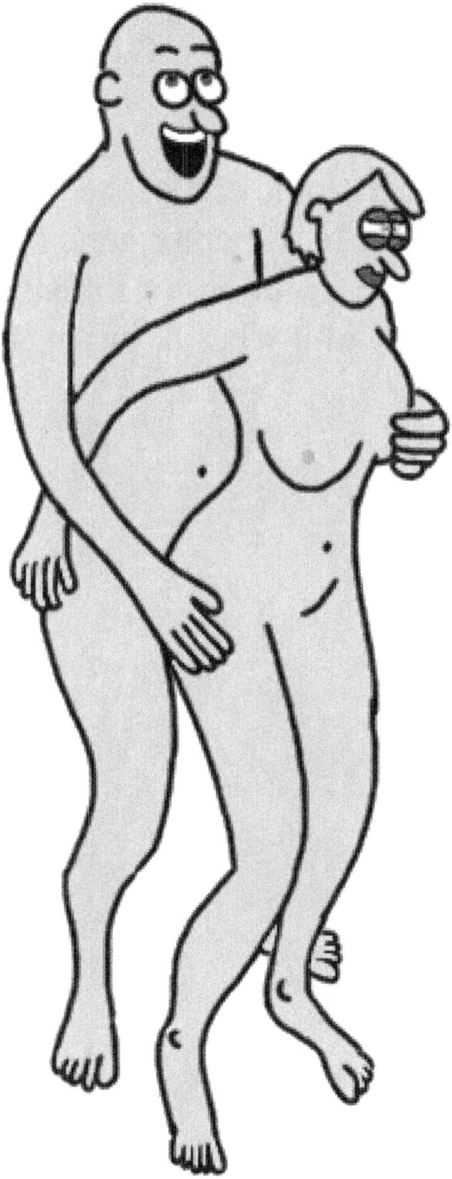

Butterfly

It's like watching two wobbling jellies on a plate, I love jelly.

Brenda lies down on the end of the bed and I kneel down between her legs. I enter her cave with my bat. Her boobies wobble with every thrust I make and I have a great view of my bat flying in and out....

Love it.

Bob

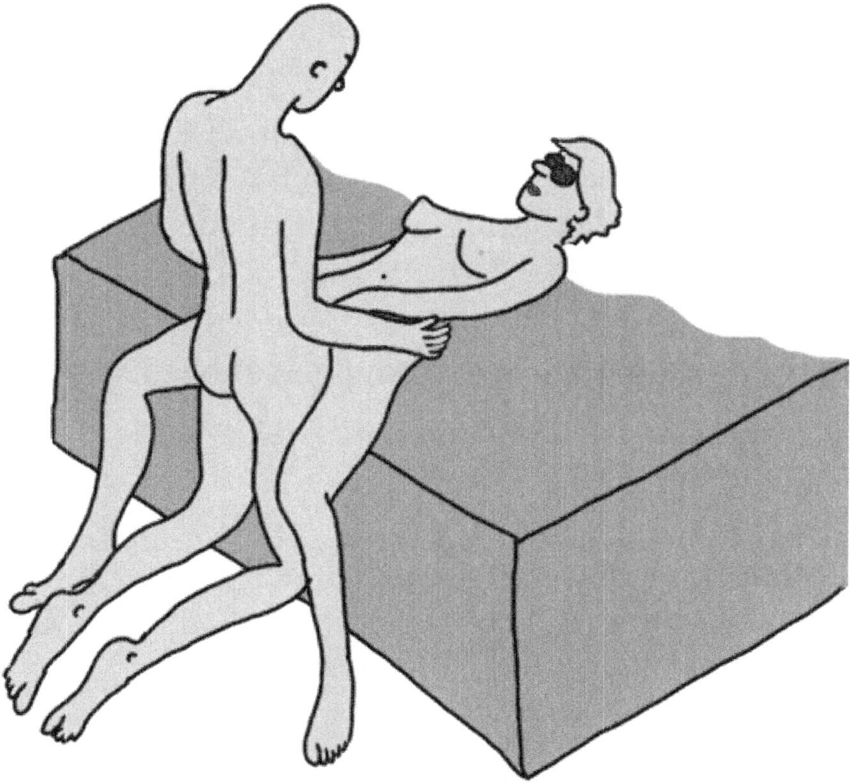

Cowboy

Ride 'em Cowboy. Bob finds this position really hard to do. He thinks his chopper is going to snap in half one day doing this position. Lol

I lie on my back and Bob lies on top of me in the Missionary position to start with. He then slowly sits upright until he is sitting on me, still keeping his chopper in my foo foo.

I love this position, everything gets rubbed.

Mmmmmm

Brenda

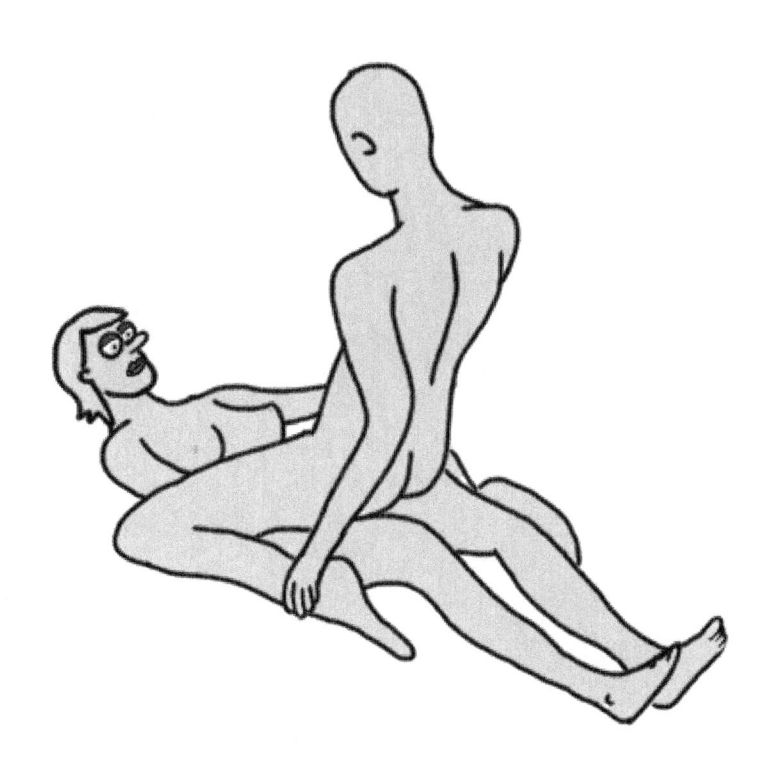

Cowgirl

My turn to Ride 'em Cowboy! Cowgirl actually.

Bob lies on the bed and I sit on his pistol.
I'm in total control with this position. I ride and grind my way to heaven. Lol

Bob's not complaining.

Brenda

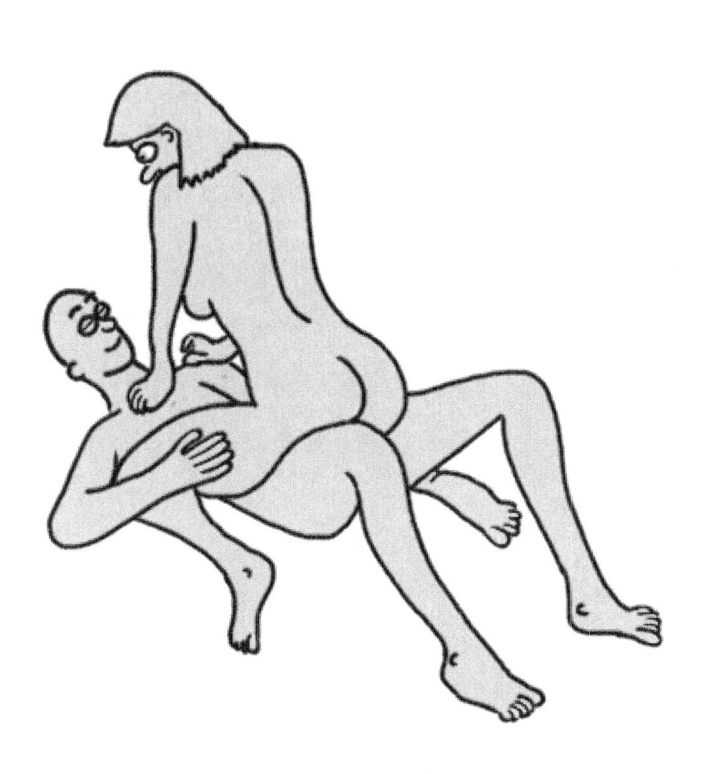

Crab

The Crab.... Crabs remind me of Brenda. She's very shellfish. Lol

This position is a natural progression from the cowgirl. Brenda just leans back and puts her feet flat on the bed. She is still in control with this one.

Love it I do.

Bob

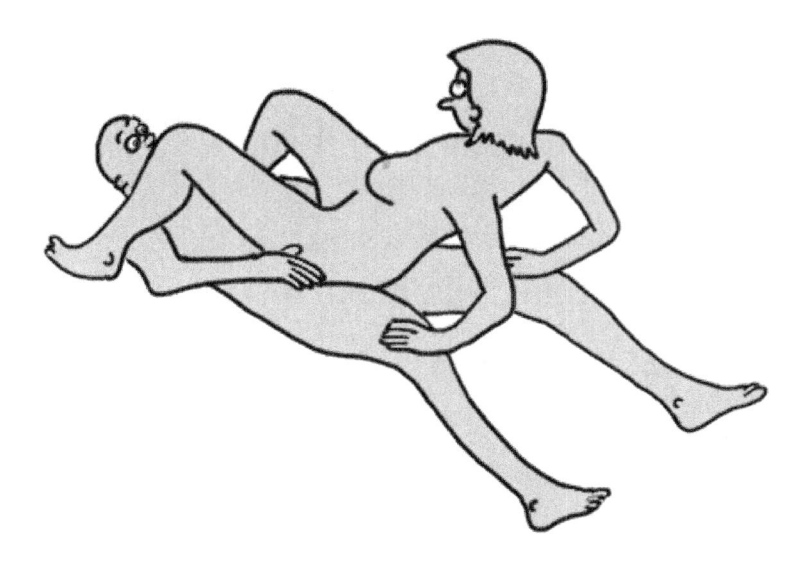

Dancer

Don't be doing this in the night clubs, unless it's an orgy party.

We stand face to face, then I wrap one leg around Bob's waist. Bob can now enter my Pom Pom with his twirler.
This is an excellent position if you want to be really passionate.

Plenty of snogging. Mmmmmm

Brenda

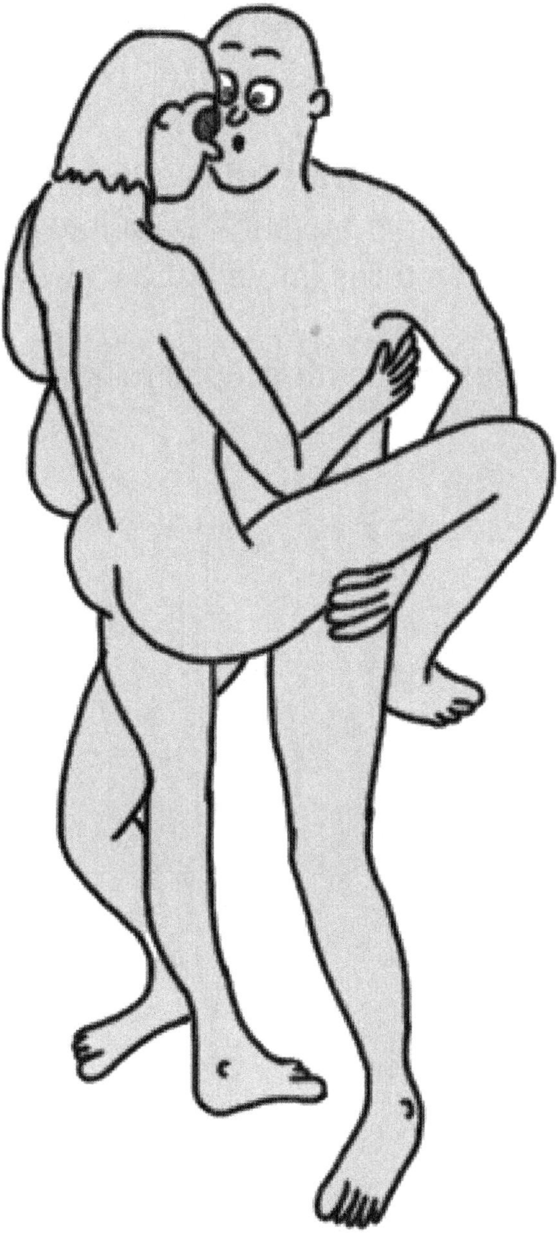

Deep Stick

If you're feeling flexible then you will love this position.

Brenda lies on her back. She lifts her legs up and rests them on my chest. I put my stick deep into her puddle. Puddle then turns into a huge wave. Lol

This is a great position with deep penetration.

Bob

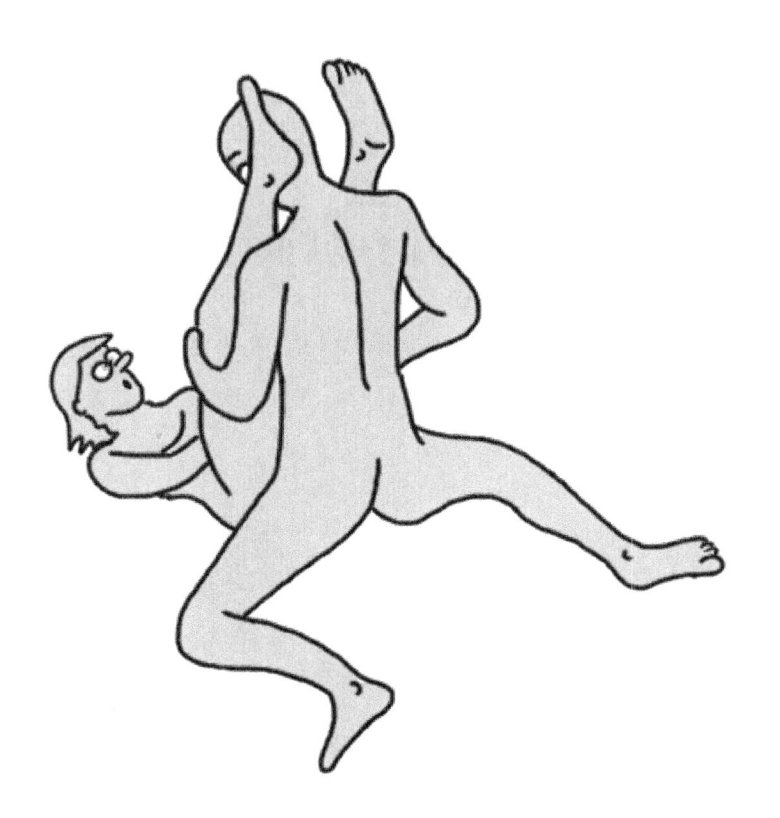

Doggy Style

Woof! Woof! Everybody knows this isn't sex with your pet pooch. That would be sick!

No, this is doing it 'like they do on the discovery channel' according to the 'Bloodhound Gang'.
Brenda is on all fours and I kneel behind her and put my Bonio into her pigs ear.
If we're feeling adventurous I put my Bonio into her pooper scooper. Lol

Bob

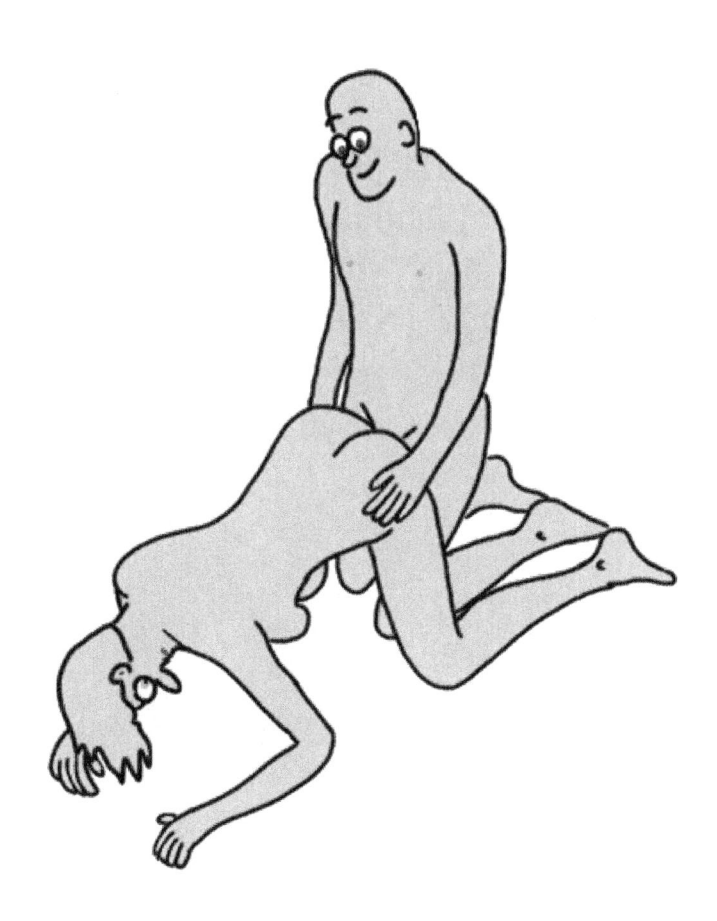

Earmuffs

The thing I like most about this position is I can call Bob every name under the sun and he can't hear me. Sometimes I'll even give my friends a ring and he has no idea. Lol

Reminds me of a headlock that I used to do when I was a member of the Llandudno wrestling club.
Bob lies on his side and I wrap my legs around his neck. He is then able to get at my tuppence with his tongue.
Loving it!

Brenda

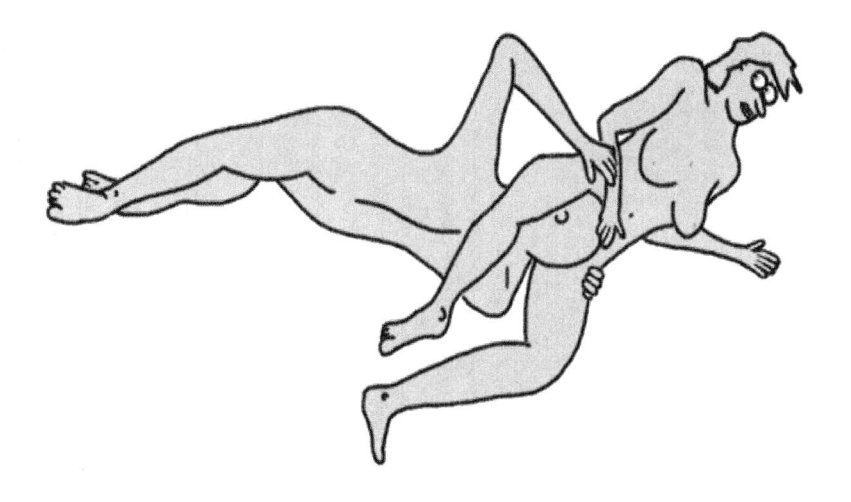

Folded Deck Chair

This is one of Brenda's favourites. I think she likes to be folded in half and treated roughly. Lol

Brenda lies on her back. Using my shoulders, I push her legs up until her knees are by her head. I can then insert my dongle into her slot.

This position is a really deep one. You might need to tie a stick to your arse.

Bob

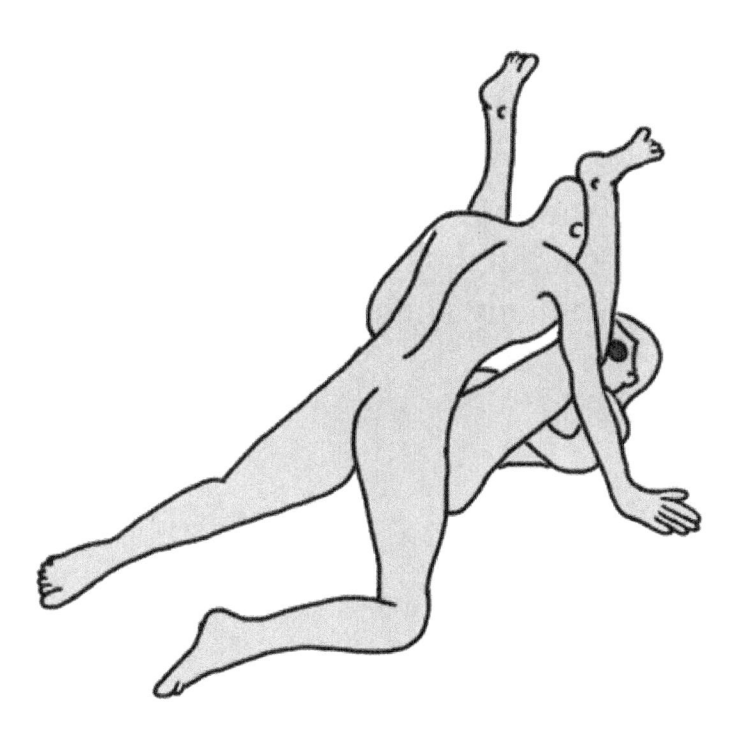

Head Rest

I've fallen asleep so many times doing his position. I'm like a baby with a dummy. Lol

It's so comfortable and Bob's leg is like a memory foam pillow. Bob gives me a slap on the side of my head when I start snoring.
It's not a boring position, but you know what it's like when you've had to many vodkas and wine.

ZZZZZZZZZZZZ

Brenda

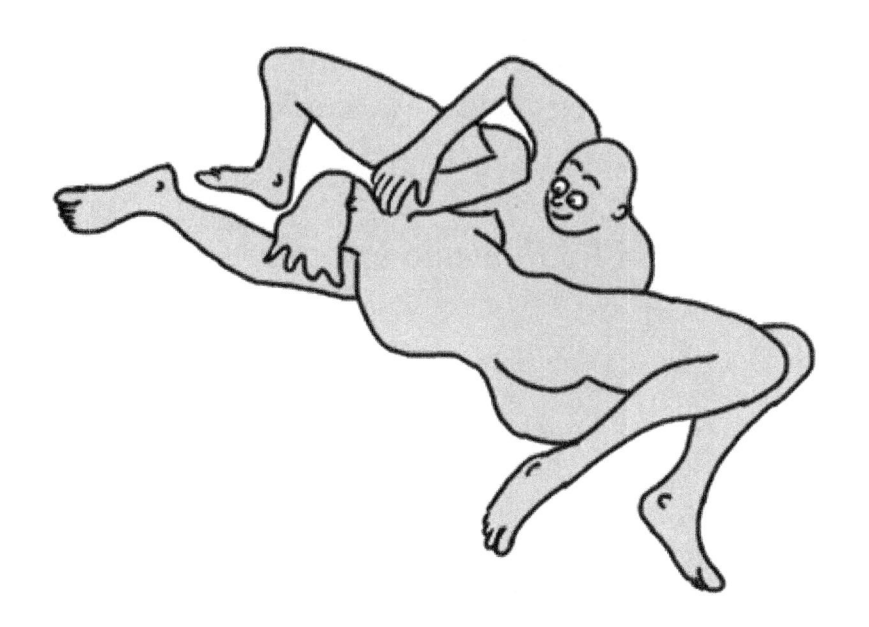

Head Rush

I love any position that puts my face in Brenda's Flip Flop. You need to be fairly fit to do this one. As long as your lady isn't a Heffalump, you should be okay.

In a standing position I hold Brenda around the waist and she puts her legs over my shoulders..

Num Num Num.
I get to eat her Flip Flop and tease her fanny nose.

Bob

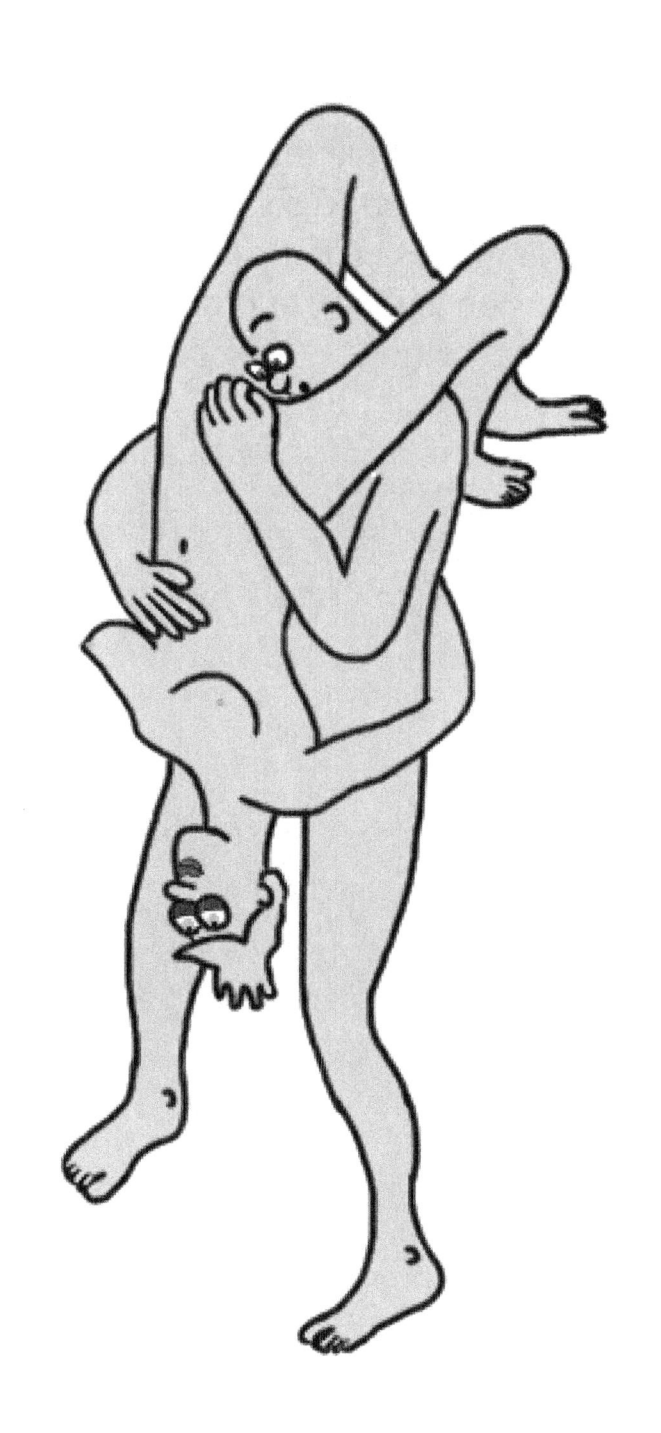

Her 68

If you're not slim like me then this is an easier alternative to the 'Head Rush' position. This is the same position but instead of standing up, we lie down. I give Bob a pillow to prop his head up and then lie back and enjoy.

I sometimes save a fart just for this position. Revenge is sweet. Lol

Brenda

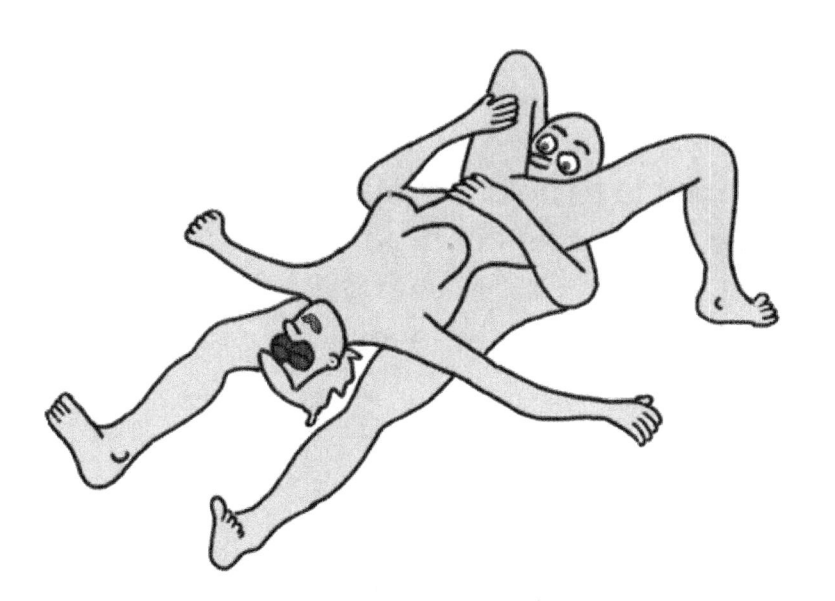

Kneeling 69

Did you know that the Chinese translation for 69 position is 'Twocanchew'? Lol

I do love a good 69 but must say that the kneeling 69 is not one of my favourite positions.
For starters, it hurts my knees unless I use my skateboarding knee pads. On the plus side, I get away with not having to hold Brenda's weight by balancing her on the floor using her head.

The things you 'chew' for love.

Bob

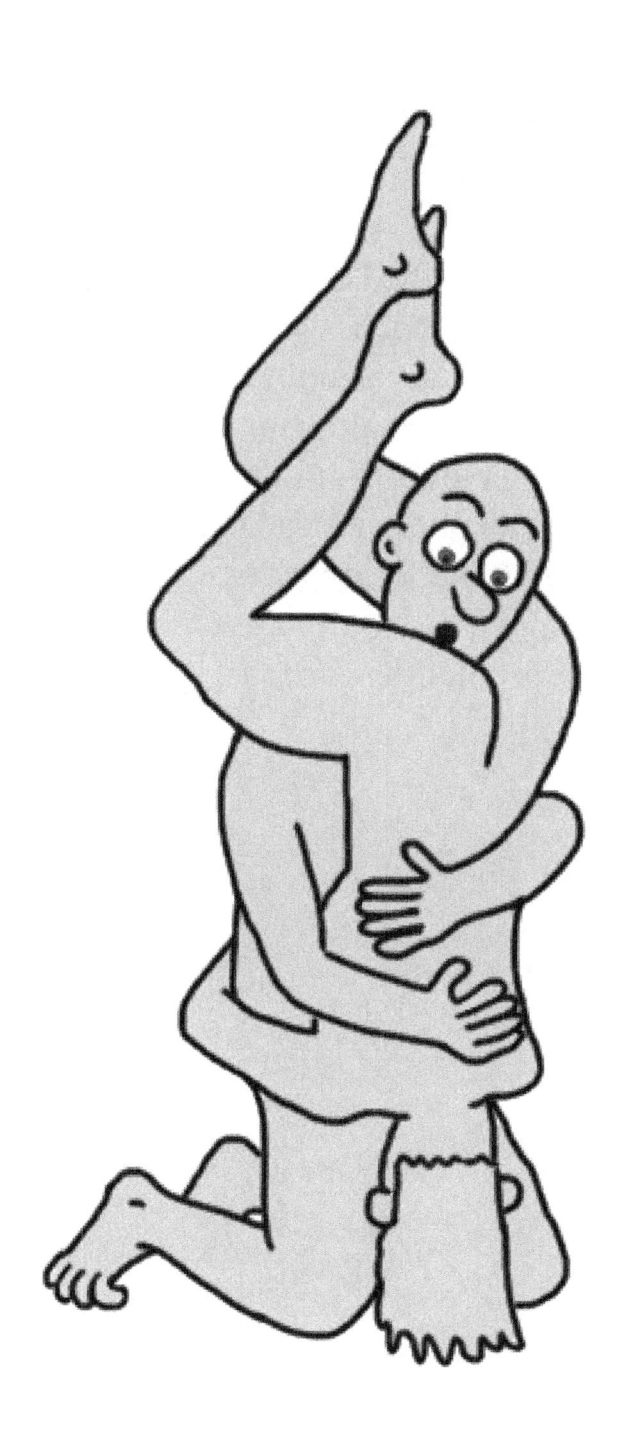

Launch Pad

I like this position, it's fun and I can get deep into Brenda's bun with my sausage.

I'll tell you why it's called the Launch Pad. When I had just started to court Brenda, we used to have sex on the lounge floor while her parents were in bed. One night we were doing this position when Brenda heard a creak coming from upstairs and thought her Dad was awake. In a panic she was able to push me off sending me flying across the room.

Houston we have a problem!!

Bob

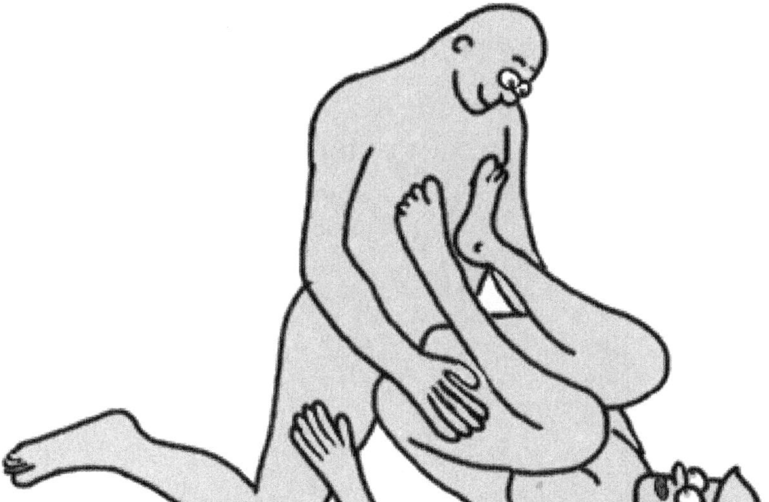

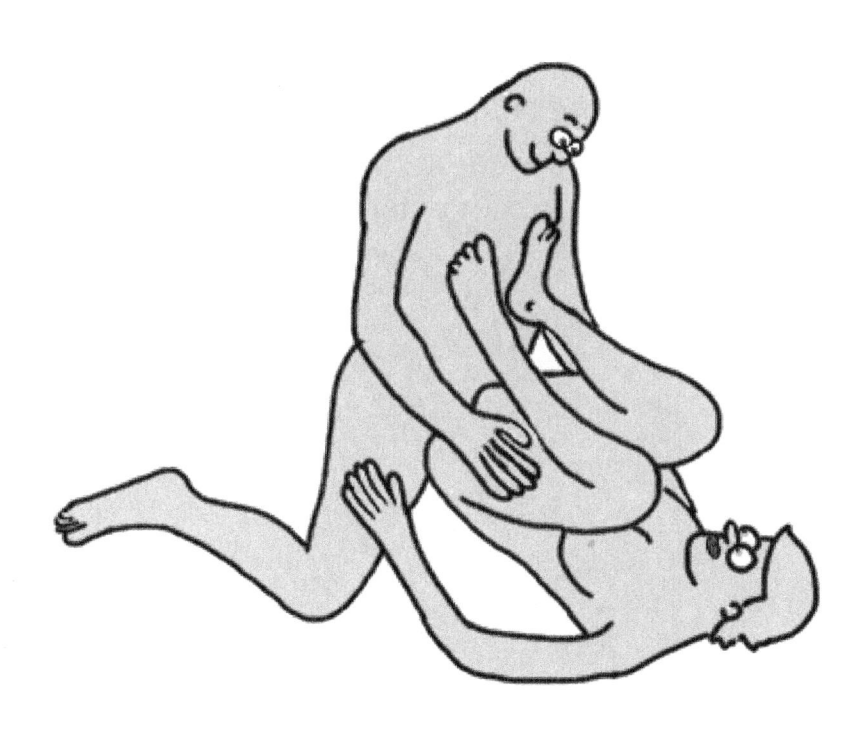

Mastery - Kneeling

Sit down and take the weight off your feet. I'll just sit on your lap and....Ooooooooh!!.

I love this position because I'm in control again and there's plenty of eye contact.
It can be done anywhere, on the sofa, office chair, end of the bed, on the loo, anywhere.

Brenda

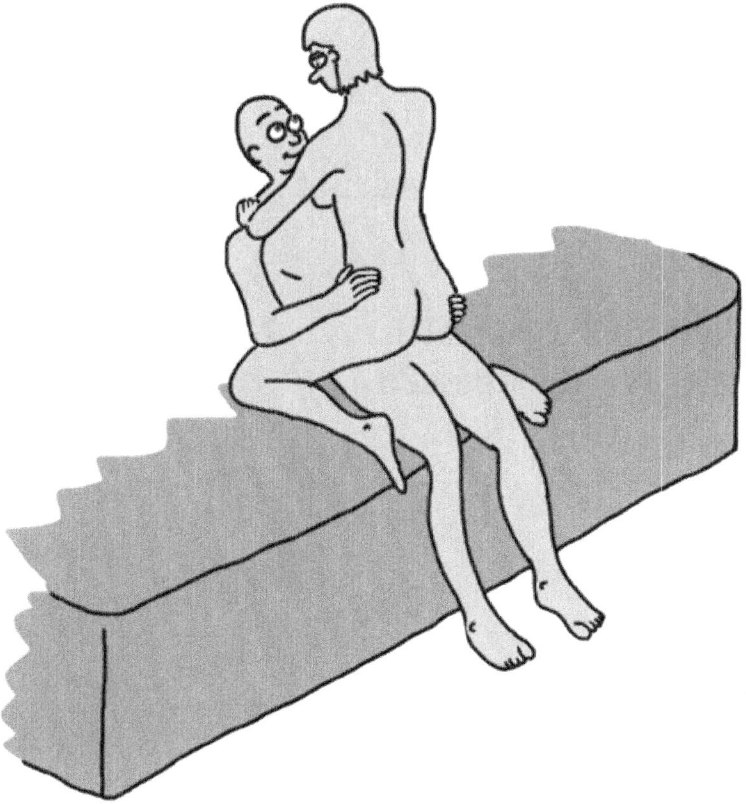

Mastery - Suspended

Feeling a bit daring? While still in the Mastery - Kneeling position you just lean right back, straighten out your legs and hey presto, it's the Mastery - Suspended position.

Make sure you get your balance right or you will slip off. Lol

Bob says he likes to watch my Jabba's wobble while doing this position. Pervert.

Brenda

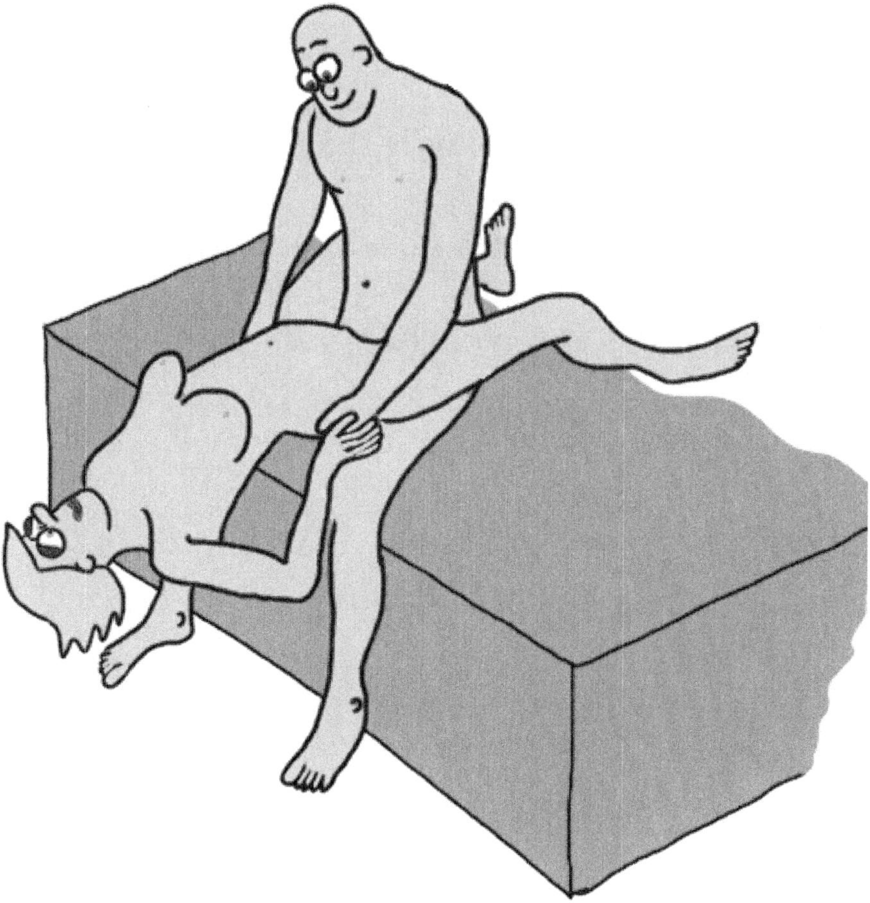

Missionary

Boring, boring, boring. I'm sorry but this position is so boring. It's the 'How you lost your virginity' position that me and Brenda no longer feel the need to do.

Two people lying down, wriggling. That's it.

Come on, get a life, be more adventurous!

Bob

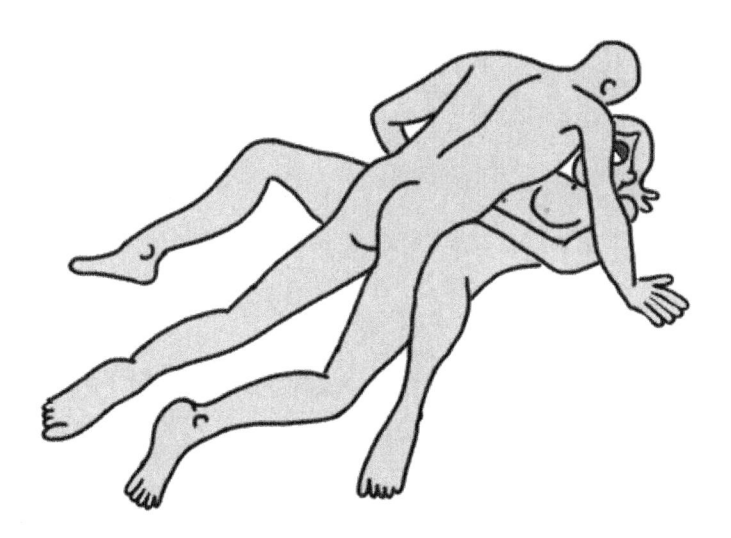

Pearly Gates

Another great position. I do love this one.

Bob lies down on the bed and I lie on top of him. My heavenly gates are open and Bob's a good man so he is allowed in.
Sometimes, I pretend he's been a bad man and send him to hell. He does love my hell hole, as long as it's been cleaned. Lol

Brenda

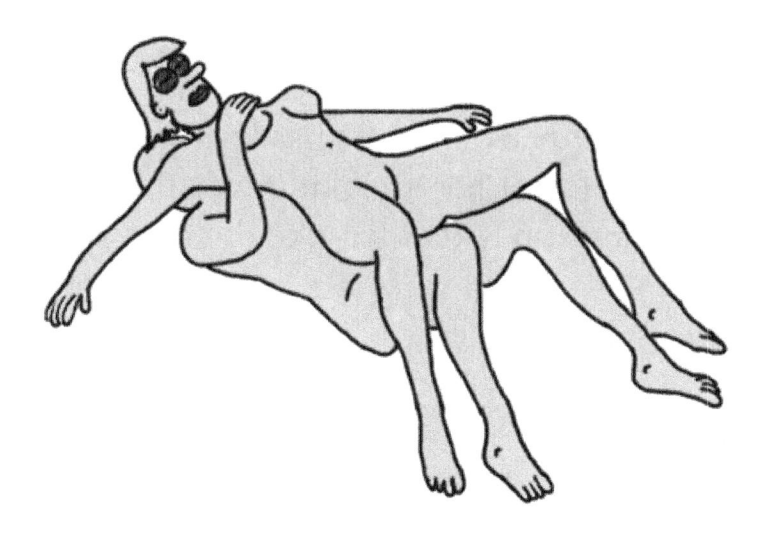

Pile Driver

My first job after leaving school was with the council. I was a road digger and I loved it. The vibration from the pneumatic drill used to get me off. You can guess why I was sacked.

This position reminds me of my council days. Brenda lies on her back and lifts her legs over her head..I then squat over her and put my drill in her manhole. I bounce up and down like I'm on a space hopper.

Bob

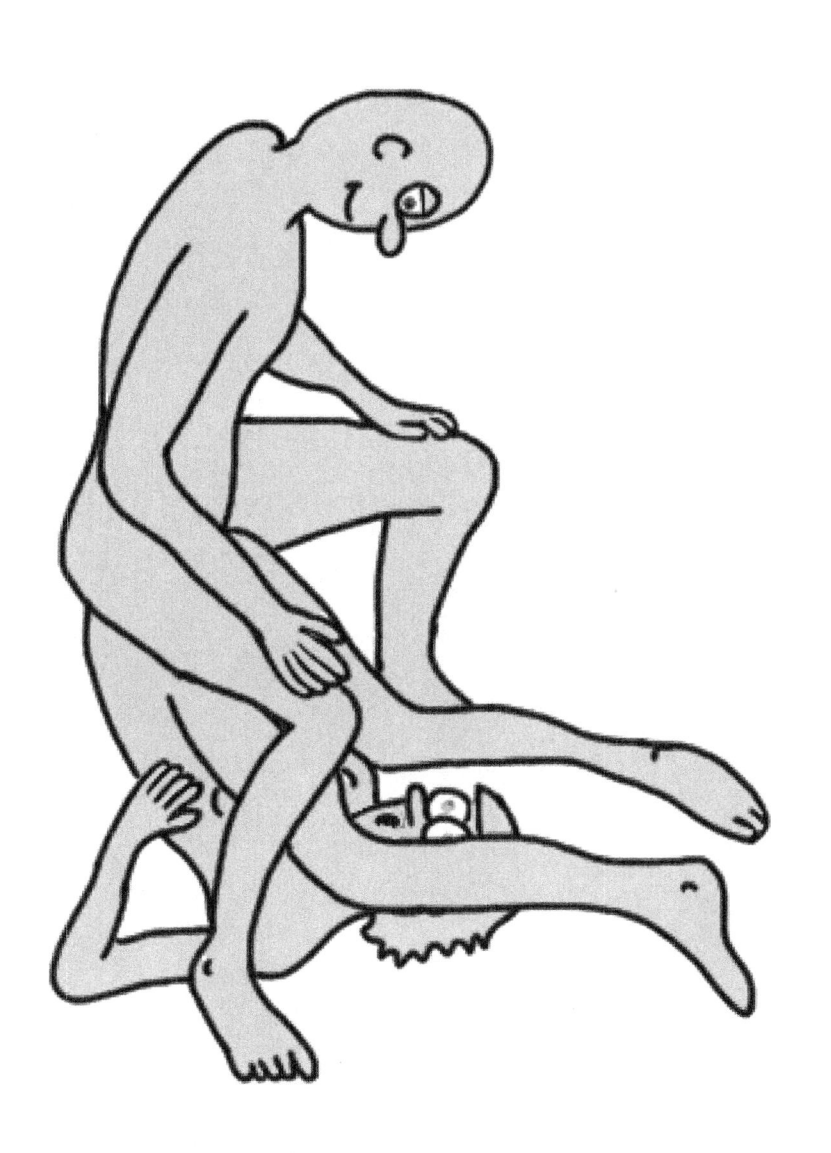

Plumber

Bob gets his Dyno Rod out for this one. My oral cavity needs a good jet clean. Lol

I lie on the bed and Bob straddles my face. I can then take his Rod in my mouth and let him clean my U-bend.

Brenda

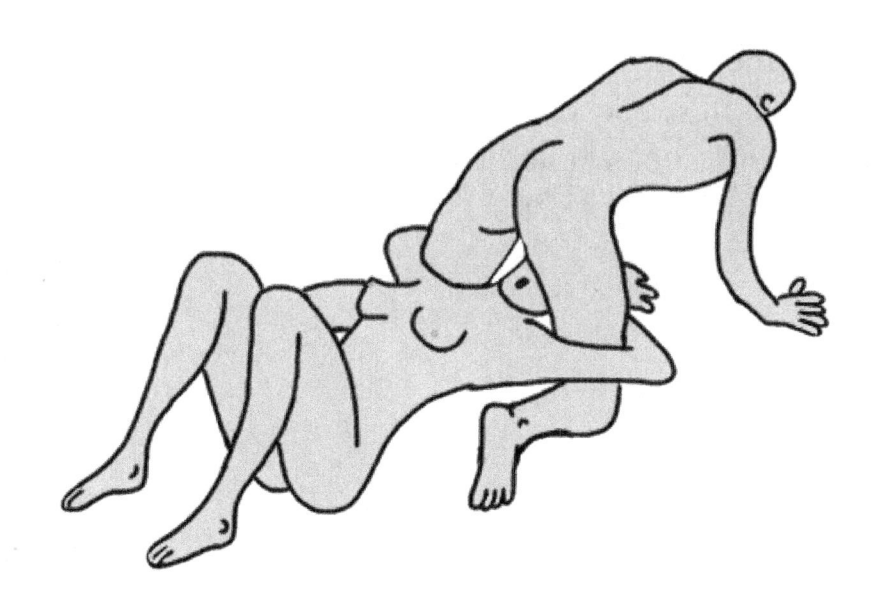

Push Cart

Did you ever do the wheelbarrow race in school? If you did then doing this position should be a piece of cake for you.

Brenda lies face down on the end of the bed with her legs over the edge. I then grab hold of her ankles and lift them up into a wheelbarrow position. I can now move closer to her whale nostril with my harpoon and spear her like Moby Dick.

Bob

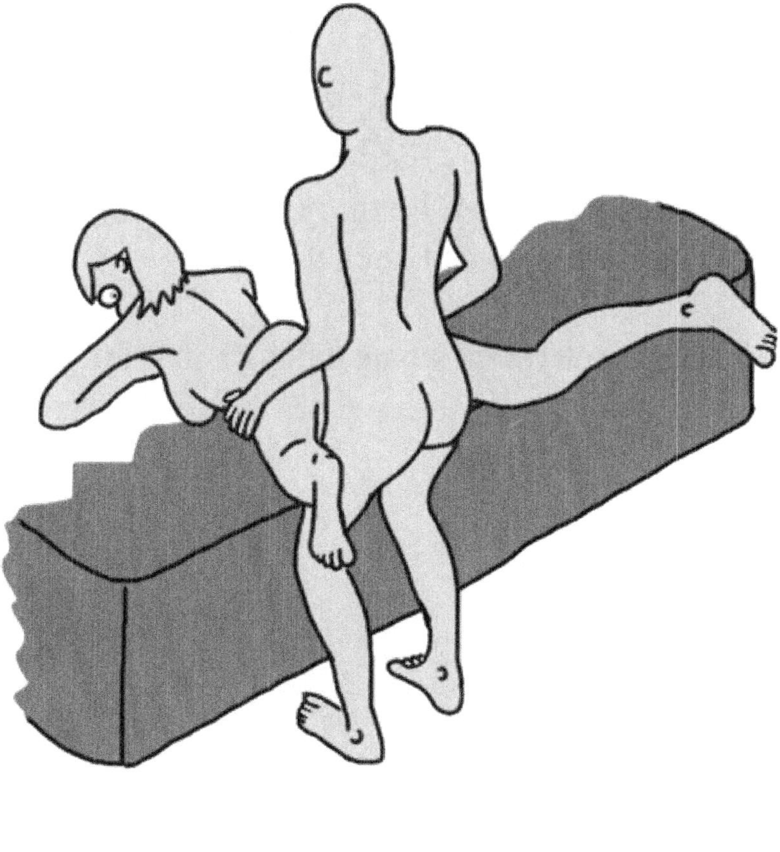

Rear Entry

Rear Entry - Entry from the rear.

There isn't a man alive who doesn't like to take his lady from the rear.
This is very similar to Doggy Style, instead of being on all fours, Brenda lies flat on her belly with her legs slightly open. I can then lie on her and put my swollen plug into her wet socket. Lol

I like to pull on Brenda's hair to show that I'm in control this time.

Bob

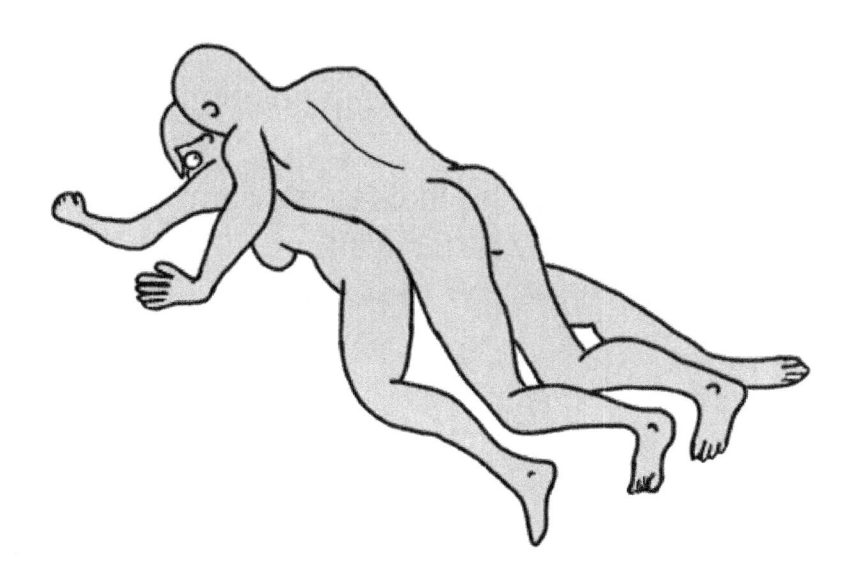

Reversed Cowgirl

This is mine and Bob's favourite position. We love it!

Bob lies on the bed and I sit on his doll's arm. I'm facing away from him as I slowly move back and forth or up and down.
I love it because it's a very deep position that reaches the parts I can't.
Bob loves it because he likes to watch my bum wobble and my brown star winking at him. Lol

Brenda

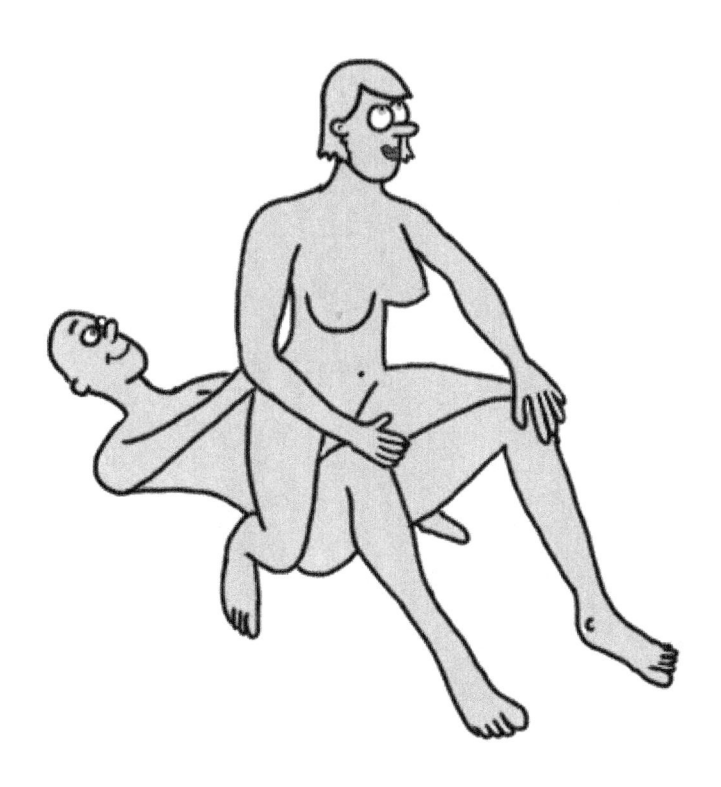

Riding Astride

Have you ever sat on the remote control by mistake? This position is very similar to that sensation.

Bob sits on the edge of the bed or sofa and I then sit on his pink remote control.
It's great with pause and rewind but don't ever fast forward!

Brenda

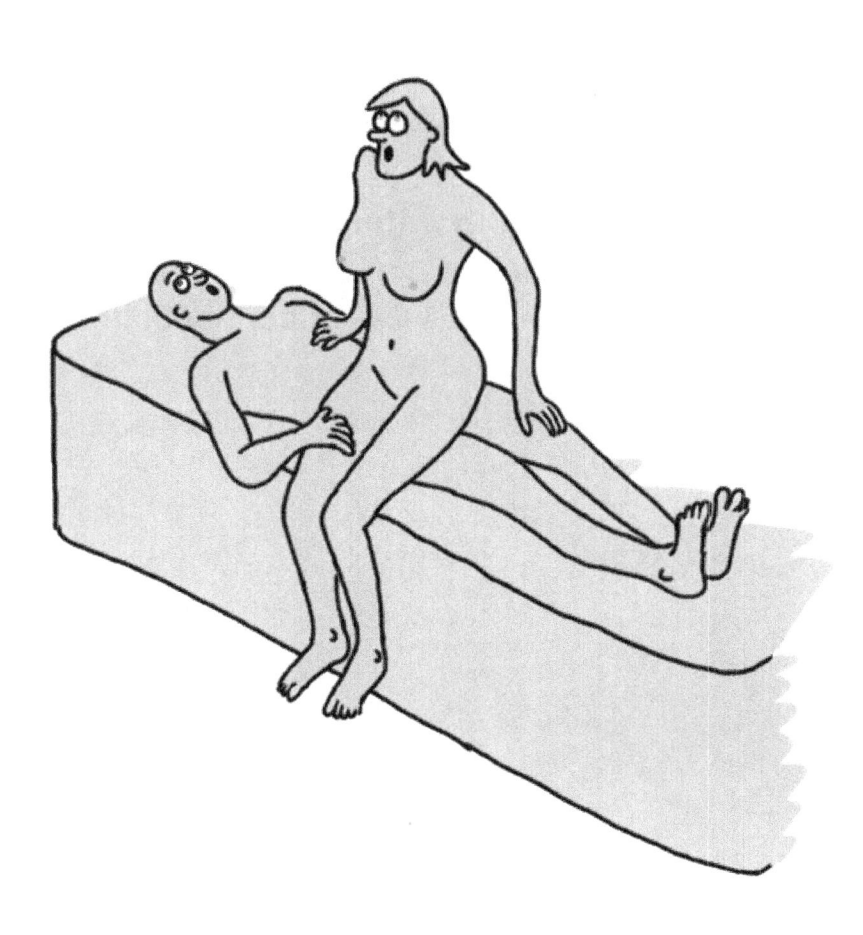

Riding The North Face

Sit on my face and tell me that you love me. Lol

When you were a kid, did your mum ever clean your face with a dirty dish cloth? She did? Then the sensation of this position won't be new to you.

Brenda cleans my face by sitting on it as I explore her dish cloth with my tongue.
It's a great feeling and the view of her big bubbles gets me in a lather.

Bob

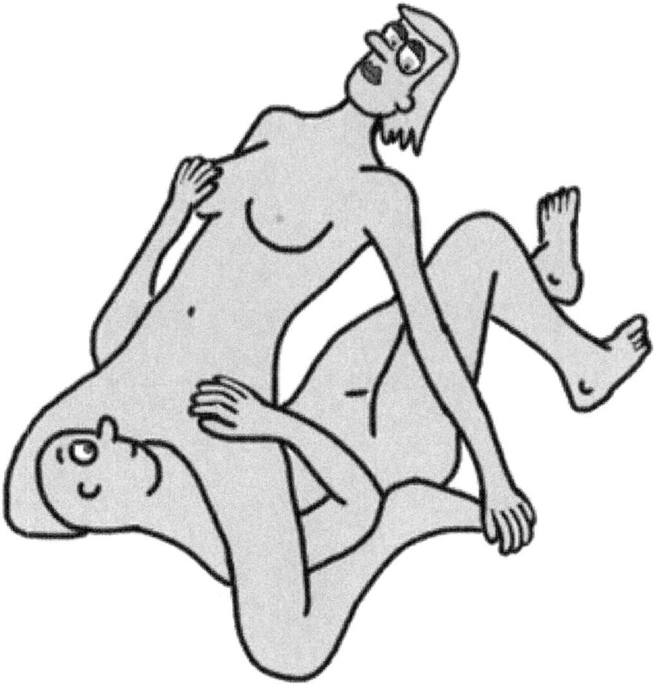

Screw

Lie on your side and pull your knees up... No, it's not my prostrate exam but another position that offers deep penetration for Brenda.

Once Brenda is in this position I just kneel by her bum and stick my thermometer up her baby tube.

Nice one!

Bob

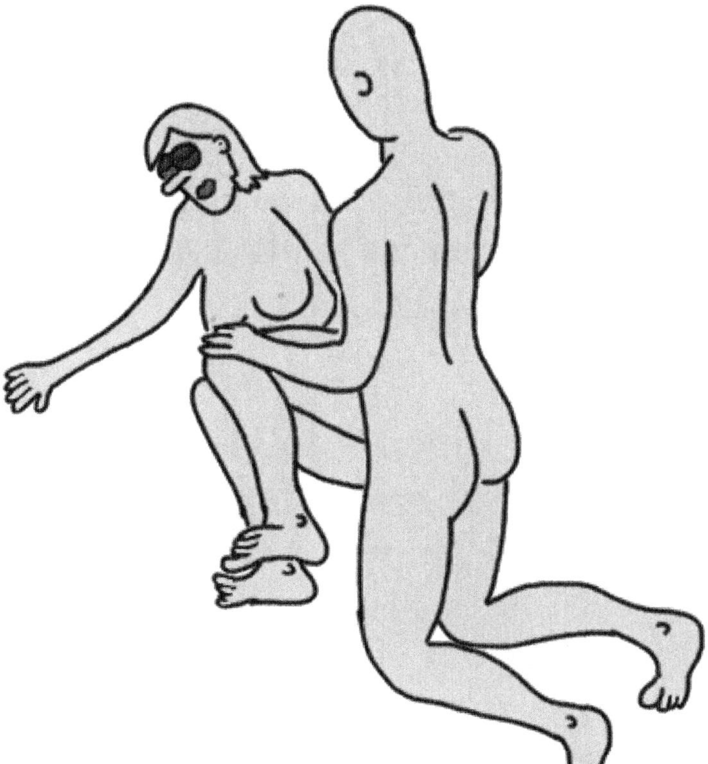

Sideways 69

What's the difference between hang gliding and oral sex? You get a better view when you are hang gliding! Lol

As with every 69 position you must make sure your bits are clean. Doing the 69 in a sideways position gives you both a leg to rest your head on.

Me and Bob can do this until we nod off. We wake up with really bad breath and a stiff neck.

Brenda

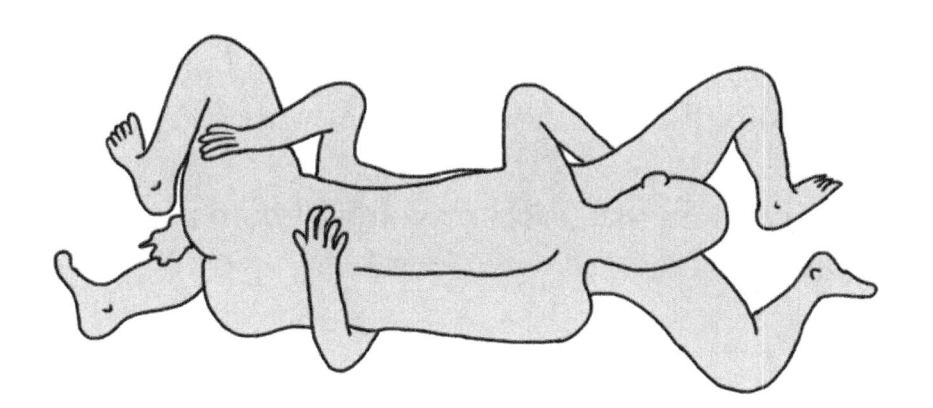

Sitting Bull

This position makes me laugh. It's so hard to thrust sitting down like this.

Brenda lies on her back and lifts her legs while I get into position.
Once her legs are on my shoulders I grab hold of her thighs and pull her towards me as I thrust.... Yee-haa!

Don't try this on the carpet or you will both get burns on your arse.

Bob

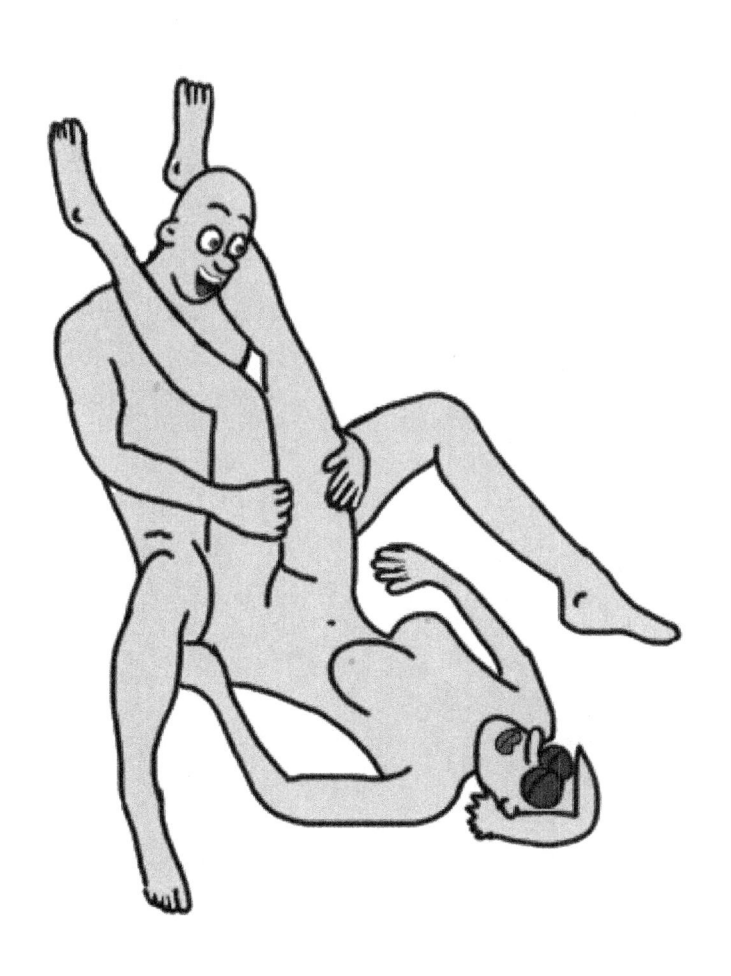

Southern Exposure

This position looks a bit mad at first but as long as Bob has had a shower and washed his bum hole I'm more than happy to do it.

Bob lies down and lifts his legs. I kneel down so I can blow his whistle and lick his plums.

Sometimes, if I'm feeling daring, I lick his bum hole too. Lol

Bob

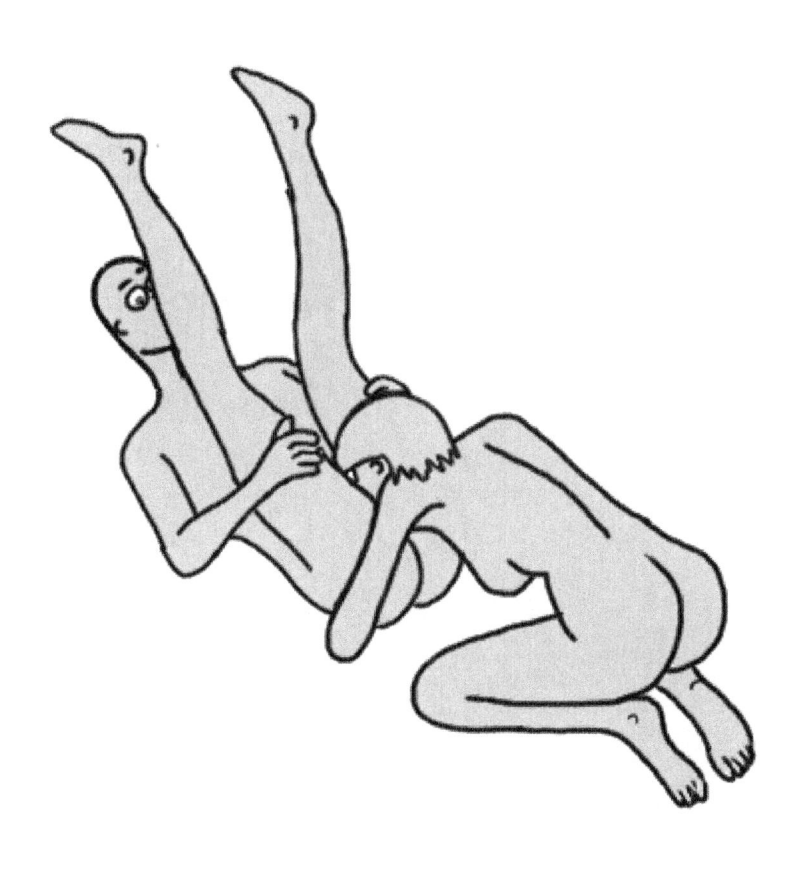

Spread Eagle

Love it, love it, love it. Anything that lets me lie down and do nothing while my numpty gets pleasured is alright by me.

I just lie back and think of Wales. Legs akimbo, Bob goes diving.

How long can Bob hold his breath? A long time. Lol

Brenda

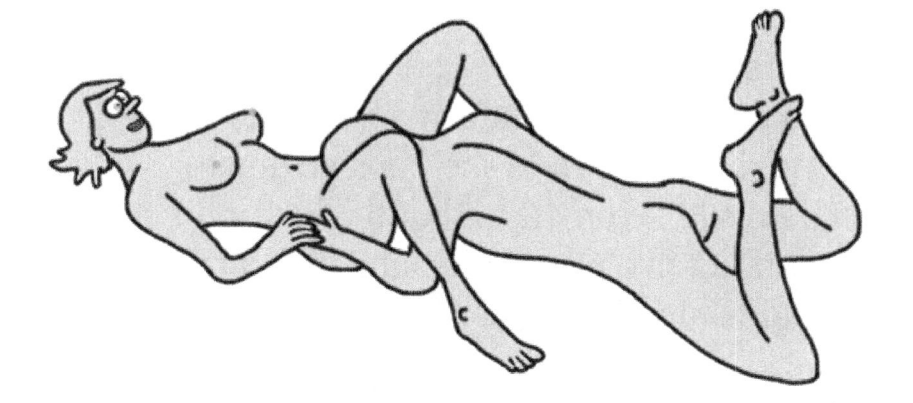

Standing 69

I have to be feeling strong to attempt this position otherwise Brenda could end up in hospital with concussion.

There are several ways to get into this position. Brenda could do a handstand against the wall and I could pick her up while she's upside down.
Brenda could lie on the end of the bed and I could lie on top of her in a 69 position and then attempt to stand up while holding her (Too difficult).

We found the best way is to start on the sofa in a 69 position and then struggle to get into a standing position. Lol

Not for the weak!

I really don't recommend doing this position. Stay well clear!

Bob

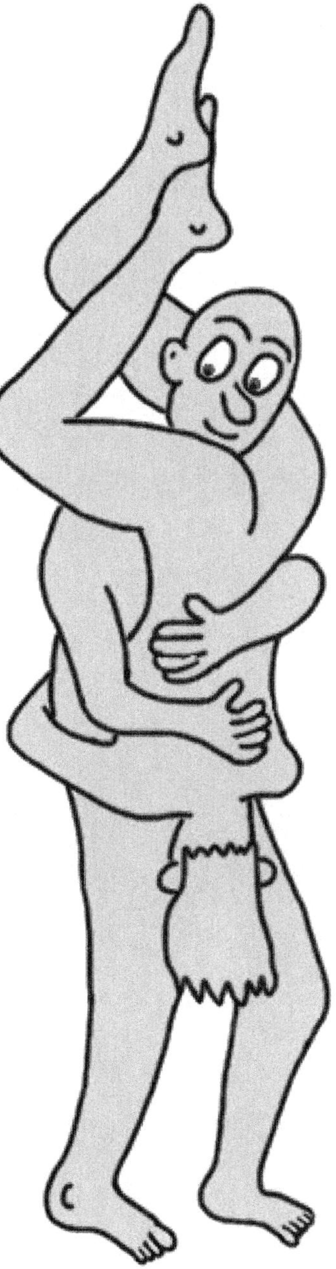

Thank you

We would like to take this opportunity to thank all our fans, worldwide.

Don't forget to visit the Bob and Brenda Joke site.

You can also find us on Face book and Twitter.

Thank you.

Printed in Great Britain
by Amazon